Good Things Come to Those Who Weight.

Realistic Affirmations for Weight Loss & Weight Management

Nutri Health & Body Company

<u>**Authors Note**</u>

All good things come with a struggle, but that doesn't mean you can't grab that struggle by the horns and enjoy the ride. Everything that happens in life is either a gift or a lesson, weight loss and weight management is both. The gift is your well-being but the lesson is what you learn along the way. No matter how hard the struggle, something good will come out of it. So remember to stay positive and embrace your journey.

Just like Ringo Starr says "Got to pay your dues if you wanna sing the blues and you know it don't come easy."

1

Health is wealth.

2

I will never give up on myself.

3

What is eaten in the dark shows in the light, so no food 3 hours before I sleep tight.

4

Exercise is a free all natural,
anti-depressant, anti-anxiety
medication.

5

Forget the word can't. Remember the word can.

6

I take care of myself because I love
myself.

7

Excuses are useless and they make one
look stupid.

8

My insecurity today will be my
confidence tomorrow.

9

I don't HAVE time to exercise, I MAKE
time.

10

I love my body.
Imperfections and all because it makes
me, Me!

11

My goal is to be healthy,
not skinny.

12

One salad won't make me lose weight.
Just like 1 doughnut won't make me fat.

13

Food is my body's friend,
not the enemy.

14

Portion control is key.

15

Don't get discouraged.
Results don't happen overnight.

16

I won't compare myself to others,
I will embrace my uniqueness.

17

Good things don't come easy.

18

Focus on health gain,
not on weight loss.

19

When I have achieved self-love,
I have achieved success.

20

I will not be hard on myself,
I am doing the best I can.

21

Don't make it a goal, make it a
lifestyle.

22

Nobody else will believe in me, if I
don't believe in myself.

23

I am exercising & eating healthy to
improve my life, not burden my life.

24

Everybody has rolls when they sit.
Skin rolls when folded.

25

A diet is temporary. A healthy
lifestyle is long term.

26

If I'm kind to my body, it will be kind to me.

27

Patience is key.

28

Overeating is abuse and will bring
nothing but regrets.

29

I eat foods that nourish my body
because I care about my body.

30

I deserve to feel good everyday.

31

Stretch marks are scars of the past,
like a wound that has healed.
Embrace them.

32

Eating smaller meals means I get to eat more often and have a faster metabolism. BONUS!

33

Everything in moderation.
Everything!

34

It takes 2 weeks for me to notice a
difference,
4 weeks for my family and 6 weeks for
everyone else.
I must be patient.

35

Like my age, the scale ain't nothin' but
a number.

36

Wine is fine but not all the time.

37

Pizza is alright as long as it's made
light.

38

One more slice of pie will go straight
to my thighs.

39

Good food can be easy, healthy and flavorful.

40

A daily herbal tea is beneficial to me.

<u>Find Me Online</u>

<u>www.nutrihbc.com</u>

Instagram: nutrihbc
Facebook: Nutri HBC

www.ingramcontent.com/pod-product-compliance
Lightning Source LLC
Chambersburg PA
CBHW031434250726
48656CB00002B/979